My Daily Tracker

DAY

DATE

FOOD DIARY

Breakfast

Lunch

Dinner

Snacks

PHYSICAL SYMPTOMS

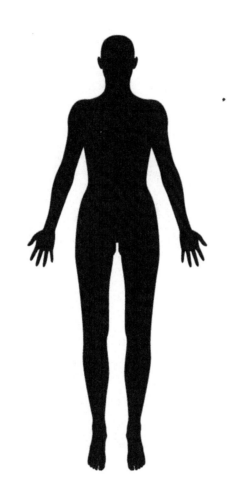

WATER   CAFFEINE   ALCOHOL

HOW I SLEPT LAST NIGHT

MOOD TRACKER

REMEMBER

My Daily Tracker

DAY

DATE

FOOD DIARY

Breakfast

Lunch

Dinner

Snacks

PHYSICAL SYMPTOMS

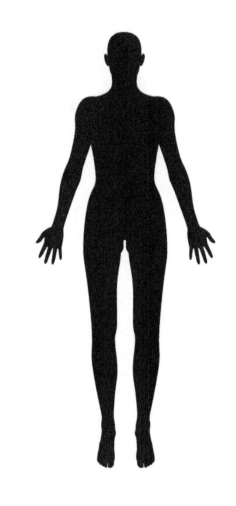

MEDICATIONS

WATER

CAFFEINE

ALCOHOL

HOW I SLEPT LAST NIGHT

MOOD TRACKER

REMEMBER

My Daily Tracker

DAY

DATE

FOOD DIARY

Breakfast

Lunch

Dinner

Snacks

PHYSICAL SYMPTOMS

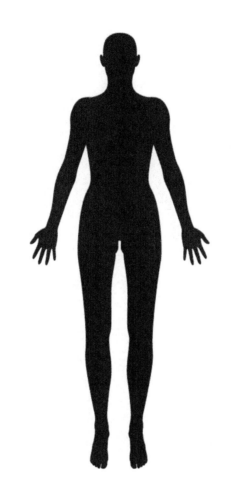

MEDICATIONS

WATER

CAFFEINE

ALCOHOL

HOW I SLEPT LAST NIGHT

MOOD TRACKER

REMEMBER

My Daily Tracker

FOOD DIARY

Breakfast

Lunch

Dinner

Snacks

PHYSICAL SYMPTOMS

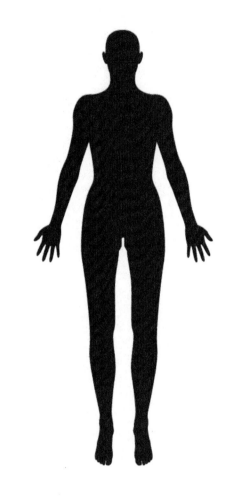

MEDICATIONS

WATER   CAFFEINE   ALCOHOL

HOW I SLEPT LAST NIGHT

MOOD TRACKER

REMEMBER

My Daily Tracker

DAY   DATE

FOOD DIARY   PHYSICAL SYMPTOMS   MEDICATIONS

Breakfast

Lunch

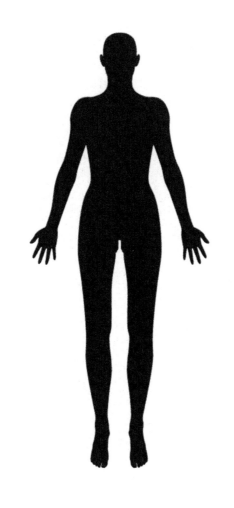

Dinner

Snacks

WATER   CAFFEINE   ALCOHOL   HOW I SLEPT LAST NIGHT   MOOD TRACKER

REMEMBER

My Daily Tracker

DAY

DATE

FOOD DIARY

Breakfast

Lunch

Dinner

Snacks

PHYSICAL SYMPTOMS

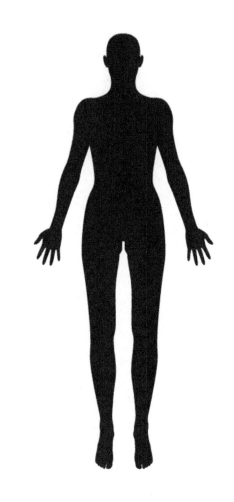

MEDICATIONS

WATER   CAFFEINE   ALCOHOL

HOW I SLEPT LAST NIGHT

MOOD TRACKER

REMEMBER

My Daily Tracker

FOOD DIARY   PHYSICAL SYMPTOMS   MEDICATIONS

Breakfast

Lunch

Dinner

Snacks

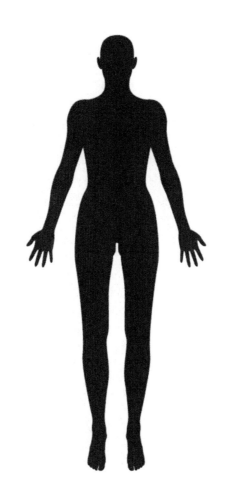

WATER   CAFFEINE   ALCOHOL   HOW I SLEPT LAST NIGHT   MOOD TRACKER

REMEMBER

My Daily Tracker

DAY

DATE

FOOD DIARY

Breakfast

Lunch

Dinner

Snacks

PHYSICAL SYMPTOMS

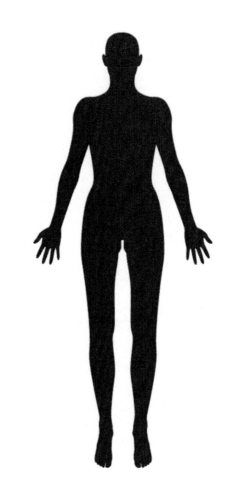

MEDICATIONS

WATER   CAFFEINE   ALCOHOL

HOW I SLEPT LAST NIGHT

MOOD TRACKER

REMEMBER

My Daily Tracker

DAY

DATE

FOOD DIARY

PHYSICAL SYMPTOMS

MEDICATIONS

Breakfast

Lunch

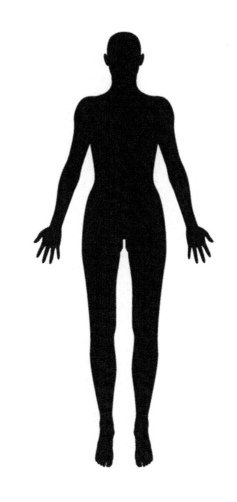

Dinner

Snacks

WATER   CAFFEINE   ALCOHOL

HOW I SLEPT LAST NIGHT

MOOD TRACKER

REMEMBER

My Daily Tracker

FOOD DIARY	PHYSICAL SYMPTOMS	MEDICATIONS

Breakfast

Lunch

Dinner

Snacks

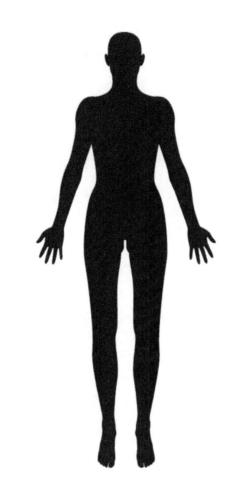

WATER	CAFFEINE	ALCOHOL	HOW I SLEPT LAST NIGHT	MOOD TRACKER

REMEMBER

My Daily Tracker

DAY

DATE

FOOD DIARY

Breakfast

Lunch

Dinner

Snacks

PHYSICAL SYMPTOMS

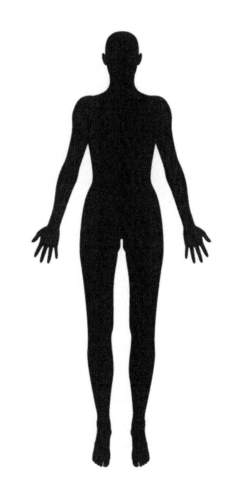

MEDICATIONS

WATER CAFFEINE ALCOHOL

HOW I SLEPT LAST NIGHT

MOOD TRACKER

REMEMBER

My Daily Tracker

DAY

DATE

FOOD DIARY

Breakfast

Lunch

Dinner

Snacks

PHYSICAL SYMPTOMS

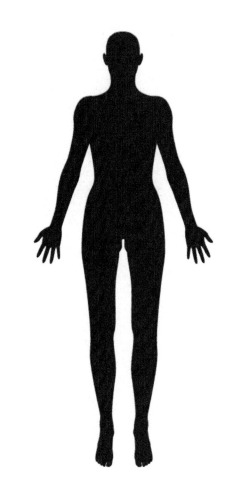

MEDICATIONS

WATER   CAFFEINE   ALCOHOL

HOW I SLEPT LAST NIGHT

MOOD TRACKER

REMEMBER

My Daily Tracker

FOOD DIARY   PHYSICAL SYMPTOMS   MEDICATIONS

Breakfast

Lunch

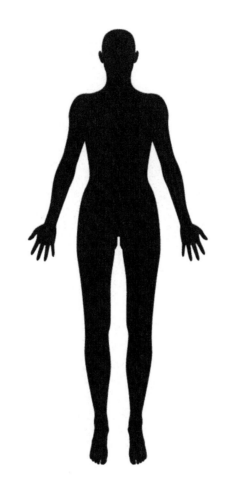

Dinner

Snacks

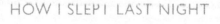

WATER   CAFFEINE   ALCOHOL   HOW I SLEPT LAST NIGHT   MOOD TRACKER

REMEMBER

My Daily Tracker

FOOD DIARY

Breakfast

Lunch

Dinner

Snacks

PHYSICAL SYMPTOMS

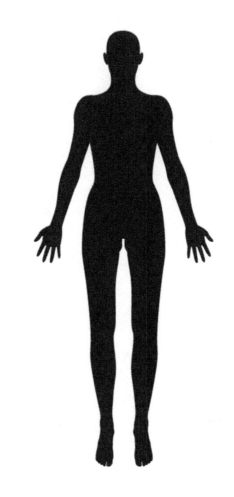

MEDICATIONS

WATER	CAFFEINE	ALCOHOL

HOW I SLEPT LAST NIGHT

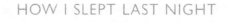

MOOD TRACKER

REMEMBER

My Daily Tracker

DAY

DATE

FOOD DIARY

Breakfast

Lunch

Dinner

Snacks

PHYSICAL SYMPTOMS

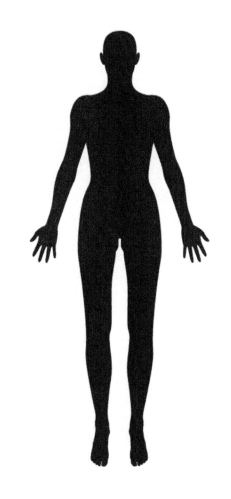

MEDICATIONS

WATER   CAFFEINE   ALCOHOL

HOW I SLEPT LAST NIGHT

MOOD TRACKER

REMEMBER

My Daily Tracker

DAY

DATE

FOOD DIARY

Breakfast

Lunch

Dinner

Snacks

PHYSICAL SYMPTOMS

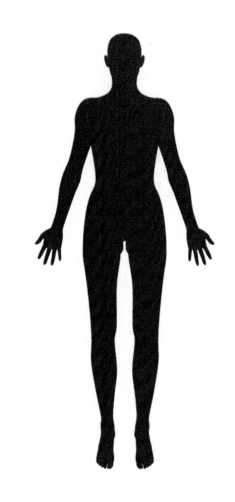

MEDICATIONS

WATER   CAFFEINE   ALCOHOL

HOW I SLEPT LAST NIGHT

MOOD TRACKER

REMEMBER

My Daily Tracker

DAY

DATE

FOOD DIARY

Breakfast

Lunch

Dinner

Snacks

PHYSICAL SYMPTOMS

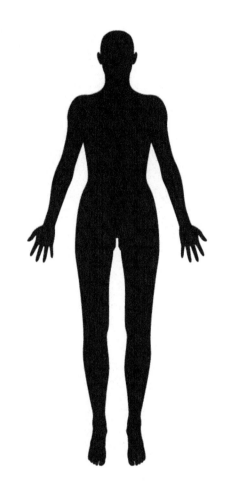

MEDICATIONS

WATER   CAFFEINE   ALCOHOL

HOW I SLEPT LAST NIGHT

MOOD TRACKER

REMEMBER

My Daily Tracker

DAY

DATE

FOOD DIARY

Breakfast

Lunch

Dinner

Snacks

PHYSICAL SYMPTOMS

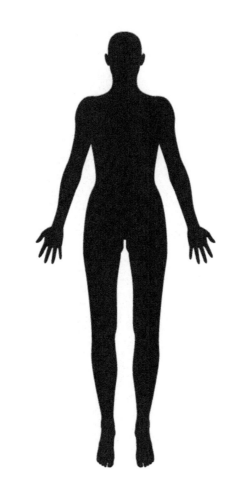

MEDICATIONS

WATER

CAFFEINE

ALCOHOL

HOW I SLEPT LAST NIGHT

MOOD TRACKER

REMEMBER

My Daily Tracker

FOOD DIARY   PHYSICAL SYMPTOMS   MEDICATIONS

Breakfast

Lunch

Dinner

Snacks

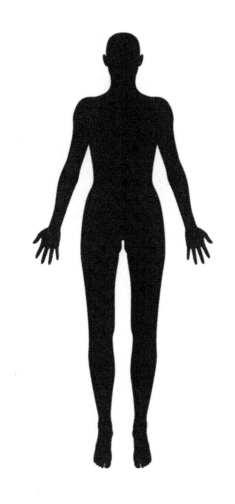

WATER   CAFFEINE   ALCOHOL   HOW I SLEPT LAST NIGHT   MOOD TRACKER

REMEMBER

My Daily Tracker

FOOD DIARY

Breakfast

Lunch

Dinner

Snacks

PHYSICAL SYMPTOMS

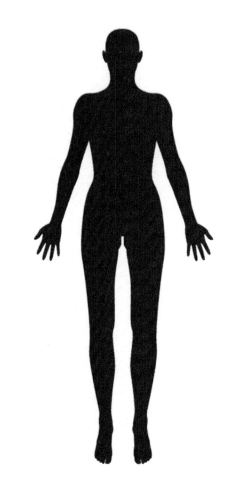

MEDICATIONS

WATER   CAFFEINE   ALCOHOL

HOW I SLEPT LAST NIGHT

MOOD TRACKER

REMEMBER

My Daily Tracker

FOOD DIARY   PHYSICAL SYMPTOMS   MEDICATIONS

Breakfast

Lunch

Dinner

Snacks

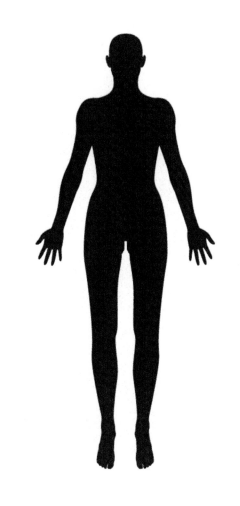

WATER   CAFFEINE   ALCOHOL   HOW I SLEPT LAST NIGHT   MOOD TRACKER

REMEMBER

My Daily Tracker

DAY   DATE

FOOD DIARY   PHYSICAL SYMPTOMS   MEDICATIONS

Breakfast

Lunch

Dinner

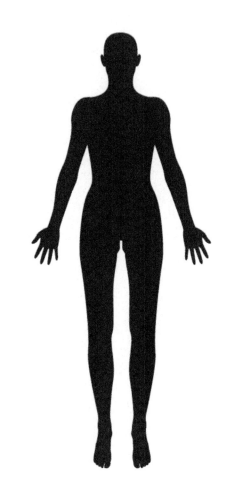

Snacks

WATER   CAFFEINE   ALCOHOL   HOW I SLEPT LAST NIGHT   MOOD TRACKER

REMEMBER

My Daily Tracker

FOOD DIARY

Breakfast

Lunch

Dinner

Snacks

PHYSICAL SYMPTOMS

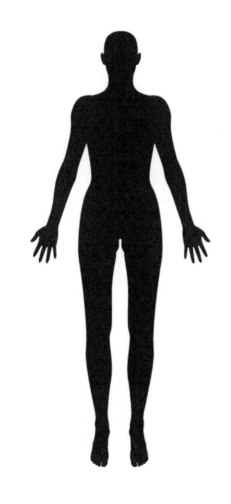

MEDICATIONS

WATER   CAFFEINE   ALCOHOL

HOW I SLEPT LAST NIGHT

MOOD TRACKER

REMEMBER

My Daily Tracker

DAY

DATE

FOOD DIARY

Breakfast

Lunch

Dinner

Snacks

PHYSICAL SYMPTOMS

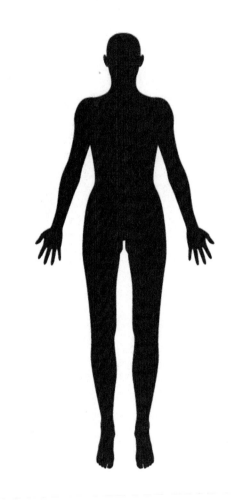

MEDICATIONS

WATER   CAFFEINE   ALCOHOL

HOW I SLEPT LAST NIGHT

MOOD TRACKER

REMEMBER

My Daily Tracker

DAY

DATE

FOOD DIARY

Breakfast

Lunch

Dinner

Snacks

PHYSICAL SYMPTOMS

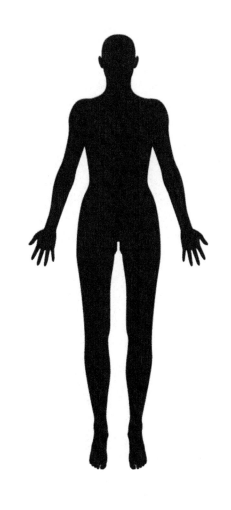

MEDICATIONS

WATER   CAFFEINE   ALCOHOL

HOW I SLEPT LAST NIGHT

MOOD TRACKER

REMEMBER

My Daily Tracker

FOOD DIARY

Breakfast

Lunch

Dinner

Snacks

PHYSICAL SYMPTOMS

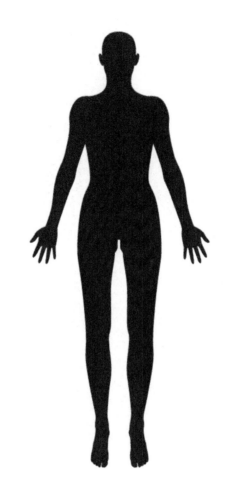

MEDICATIONS

WATER   CAFFEINE   ALCOHOL

HOW I SLEPT LAST NIGHT

MOOD TRACKER

REMEMBER

My Daily Tracker

DAY

DATE

FOOD DIARY

Breakfast

Lunch

Dinner

Snacks

PHYSICAL SYMPTOMS

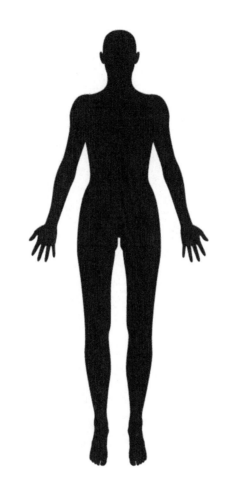

MEDICATIONS

WATER   CAFFEINE   ALCOHOL

HOW I SLEPT LAST NIGHT

MOOD TRACKER

REMEMBER

My Daily Tracker

FOOD DIARY	PHYSICAL SYMPTOMS	MEDICATIONS

Breakfast

Lunch

Dinner

Snacks

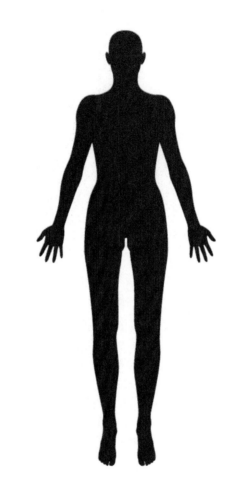

WATER	CAFFEINE	ALCOHOL	HOW I SLEPT LAST NIGHT	MOOD TRACKER

REMEMBER

My Daily Tracker

FOOD DIARY   PHYSICAL SYMPTOMS   MEDICATIONS

Breakfast

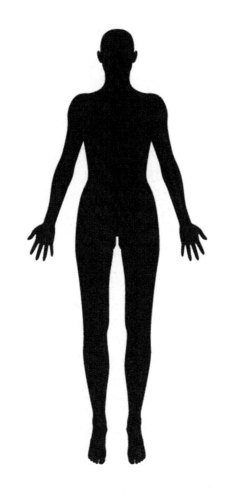

Lunch

Dinner

Snacks

WATER   CAFFEINE   ALCOHOL   HOW I SLEPT LAST NIGHT   MOOD TRACKER

REMEMBER

My Daily Tracker

FOOD DIARY	PHYSICAL SYMPTOMS	MEDICATIONS

Breakfast

Lunch

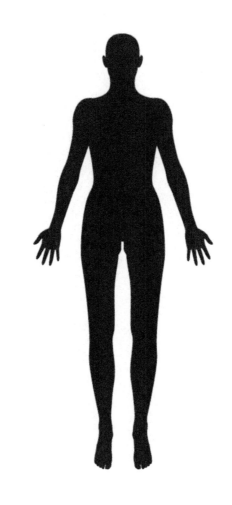

Dinner

Snacks

WATER   CAFFEINE   ALCOHOL   HOW I SLEPT LAST NIGHT   MOOD TRACKER

REMEMBER

My Daily Tracker

DAY

DATE

FOOD DIARY

Breakfast

Lunch

Dinner

Snacks

PHYSICAL SYMPTOMS

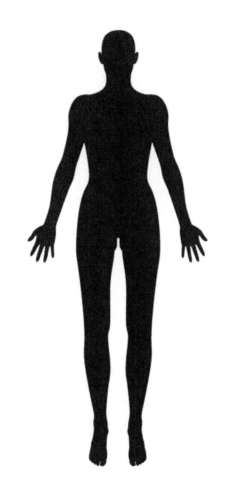

MEDICATIONS

WATER   CAFFEINE   ALCOHOL

HOW I SLEPT LAST NIGHT

MOOD TRACKER

REMEMBER

My Daily Tracker

DAY   DATE

FOOD DIARY   ## PHYSICAL SYMPTOMS   ## MEDICATIONS

Breakfast

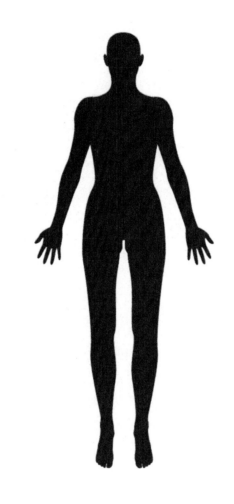

Lunch

Dinner

Snacks

WATER   CAFFEINE   ALCOHOL   HOW I SLEPT LAST NIGHT   MOOD TRACKER

REMEMBER

My Daily Tracker

DAY

DATE

FOOD DIARY

Breakfast

Lunch

Dinner

Snacks

PHYSICAL SYMPTOMS

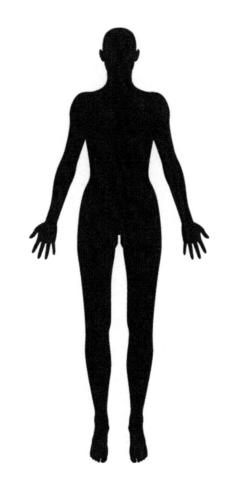

MEDICATIONS

WATER   CAFFEINE   ALCOHOL

HOW I SLEPT LAST NIGHT

MOOD TRACKER

REMEMBER

My Daily Tracker

DAY

DATE

FOOD DIARY

Breakfast

Lunch

Dinner

Snacks

PHYSICAL SYMPTOMS

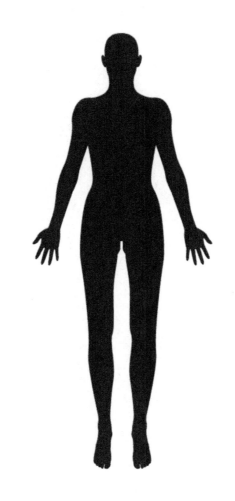

MEDICATIONS

WATER   CAFFEINE   ALCOHOL

HOW I SLEPT LAST NIGHT

MOOD TRACKER

REMEMBER

My Daily Tracker

DAY

DATE

FOOD DIARY

PHYSICAL SYMPTOMS

MEDICATIONS

Breakfast

Lunch

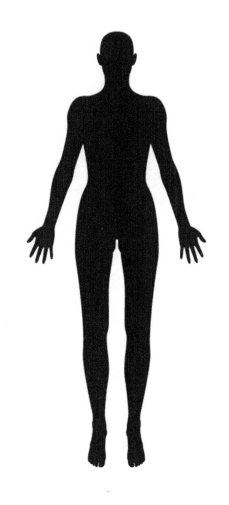

Dinner

Snacks

WATER CAFFEINE ALCOHOL

HOW I SLEPT LAST NIGHT

MOOD TRACKER

REMEMBER

My Daily Tracker

DAY

DATE

FOOD DIARY

Breakfast

Lunch

Dinner

Snacks

PHYSICAL SYMPTOMS

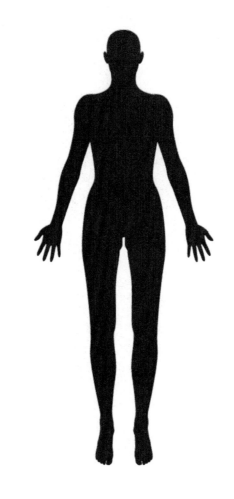

MEDICATIONS

WATER

CAFFEINE

ALCOHOL

HOW I SLEPT LAST NIGHT

MOOD TRACKER

REMEMBER

My Daily Tracker

DAY

DATE

FOOD DIARY

Breakfast

Lunch

Dinner

Snacks

PHYSICAL SYMPTOMS

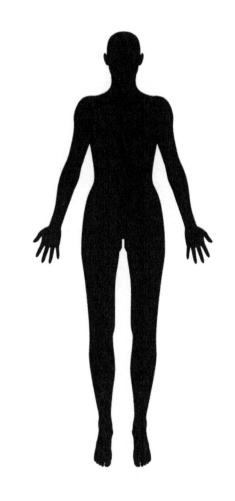

MEDICATIONS

WATER CAFFEINE ALCOHOL

HOW I SLEPT LAST NIGHT

MOOD TRACKER

REMEMBER

My Daily Tracker

DAY   DATE

FOOD DIARY

Breakfast

Lunch

Dinner

Snacks

PHYSICAL SYMPTOMS

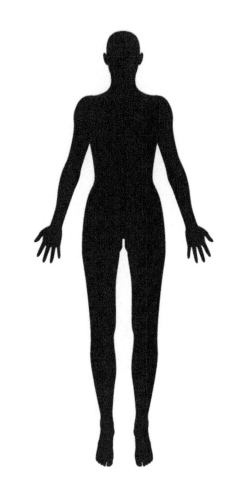

MEDICATIONS

WATER   CAFFEINE   ALCOHOL

HOW I SLEPT LAST NIGHT

MOOD TRACKER

REMEMBER

My Daily Tracker

DAY

DATE

FOOD DIARY

PHYSICAL SYMPTOMS

MEDICATIONS

Breakfast

Lunch

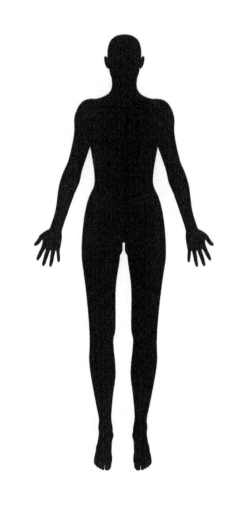

Dinner

Snacks

WATER   CAFFEINE   ALCOHOL

HOW I SLEPT LAST NIGHT

MOOD TRACKER

REMEMBER

My Daily Tracker

FOOD DIARY PHYSICAL SYMPTOMS MEDICATIONS

Breakfast

Lunch

Dinner

Snacks

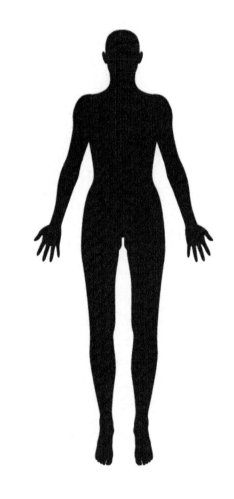

WATER CAFFEINE ALCOHOL HOW I SLEPT LAST NIGHT MOOD TRACKER

REMEMBER

My Daily Tracker

DAY

DATE

FOOD DIARY

PHYSICAL SYMPTOMS

MEDICATIONS

Breakfast

Lunch

Dinner

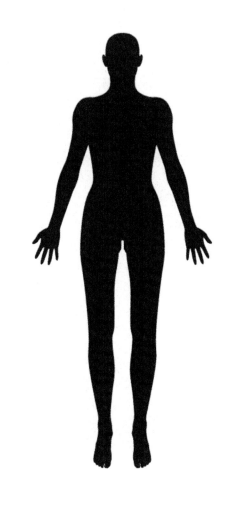

Snacks

WATER   CAFFEINE   ALCOHOL   HOW I SLEPT LAST NIGHT   MOOD TRACKER

REMEMBER

My Daily Tracker

FOOD DIARY   PHYSICAL SYMPTOMS   MEDICATIONS

Breakfast

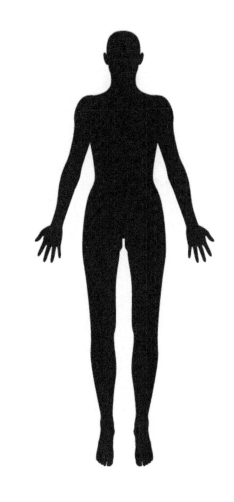

Lunch

Dinner

Snacks

WATER   CAFFEINE   ALCOHOL   HOW I SLEPT LAST NIGHT   MOOD TRACKER

REMEMBER

My Daily Tracker

DAY

DATE

FOOD DIARY

PHYSICAL SYMPTOMS

MEDICATIONS

Breakfast

Lunch

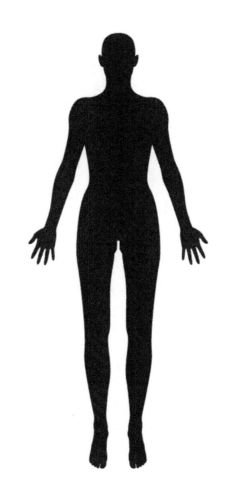

Dinner

Snacks

WATER

CAFFEINE

ALCOHOL

HOW I SLEPT LAST NIGHT

MOOD TRACKER

REMEMBER

My Daily Tracker

FOOD DIARY

Breakfast

Lunch

Dinner

Snacks

PHYSICAL SYMPTOMS

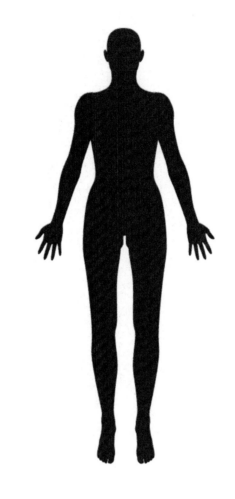

MEDICATIONS

WATER   CAFFEINE   ALCOHOL

HOW I SLEPT LAST NIGHT

MOOD TRACKER

REMEMBER

My Daily Tracker

FOOD DIARY   PHYSICAL SYMPTOMS   MEDICATIONS

Breakfast

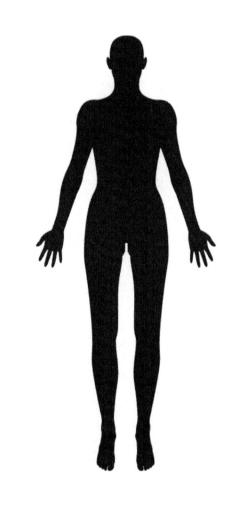

Lunch

Dinner

Snacks

WATER   CAFFEINE   ALCOHOL   HOW I SLEPT LAST NIGHT   MOOD TRACKER

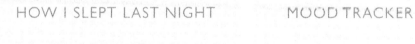

REMEMBER

My Daily Tracker

DAY

DATE

FOOD DIARY

Breakfast

Lunch

Dinner

Snacks

PHYSICAL SYMPTOMS

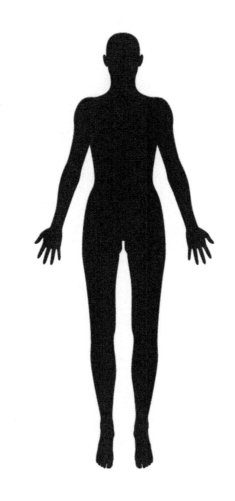

MEDICATIONS

WATER	CAFFEINE	ALCOHOL

HOW I SLEPT LAST NIGHT

MOOD TRACKER

REMEMBER

My Daily Tracker

DAY

DATE

FOOD DIARY

Breakfast

Lunch

Dinner

Snacks

PHYSICAL SYMPTOMS

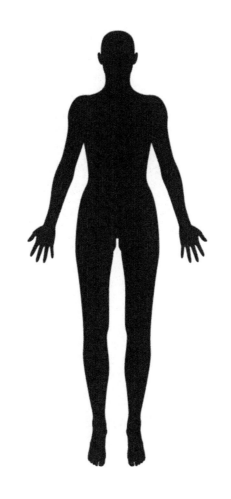

MEDICATIONS

WATER

CAFFEINE

ALCOHOL

HOW I SLEPT LAST NIGHT

MOOD TRACKER

REMEMBER

My Daily Tracker

DAY

DATE

FOOD DIARY

Breakfast

Lunch

Dinner

Snacks

PHYSICAL SYMPTOMS

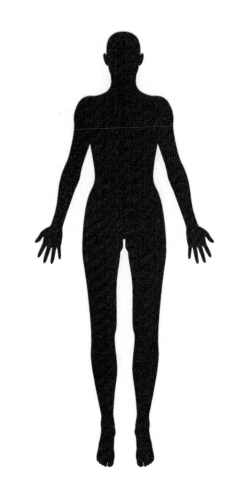

MEDICATIONS

WATER

CAFFEINE

ALCOHOL

HOW I SLEPT LAST NIGHT

MOOD TRACKER

REMEMBER

My Daily Tracker

FOOD DIARY

PHYSICAL SYMPTOMS

MEDICATIONS

Breakfast

Lunch

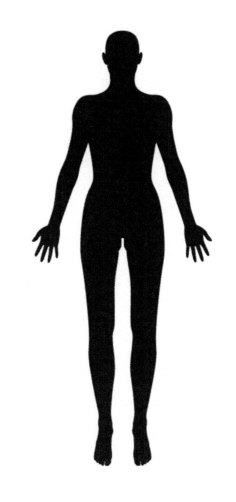

Dinner

Snacks

WATER CAFFEINE ALCOHOL

HOW I SLEPT LAST NIGHT

MOOD TRACKER

REMEMBER

My Daily Tracker

DAY

DATE

FOOD DIARY

Breakfast

Lunch

Dinner

Snacks

PHYSICAL SYMPTOMS

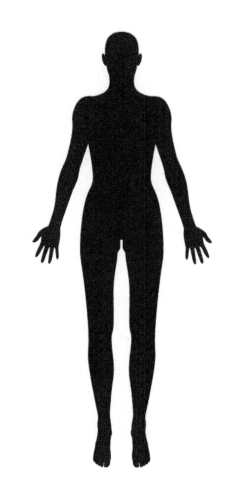

MEDICATIONS

WATER   CAFFEINE   ALCOHOL

HOW I SLEPT LAST NIGHT

MOOD TRACKER

REMEMBER

My Daily Tracker

DAY

DATE

FOOD DIARY

Breakfast

Lunch

Dinner

Snacks

PHYSICAL SYMPTOMS

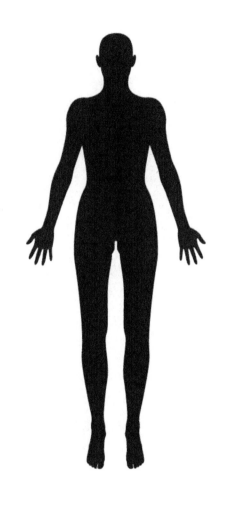

MEDICATIONS

WATER CAFFEINE ALCOHOL

HOW I SLEPT LAST NIGHT

MOOD TRACKER

REMEMBER

My Daily Tracker

DAY

DATE

FOOD DIARY	PHYSICAL SYMPTOMS	MEDICATIONS

Breakfast

Lunch

Dinner

Snacks

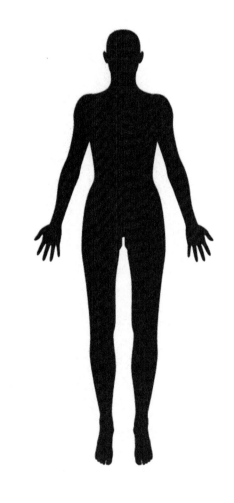

WATER	CAFFEINE	ALCOHOL	HOW I SLEPT LAST NIGHT	MOOD TRACKER

REMEMBER

My Daily Tracker

DAY

DATE

FOOD DIARY

Breakfast

Lunch

Dinner

Snacks

PHYSICAL SYMPTOMS

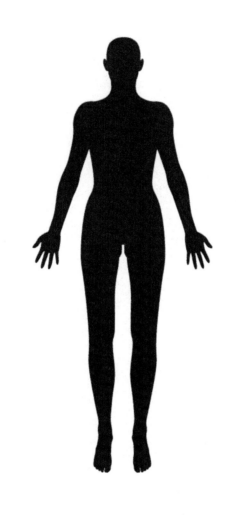

MEDICATIONS

WATER   CAFFEINE   ALCOHOL

HOW I SLEPT LAST NIGHT

MOOD TRACKER

REMEMBER

My Daily Tracker

DAY

DATE

FOOD DIARY

PHYSICAL SYMPTOMS

MEDICATIONS

Breakfast

Lunch

Dinner

Snacks

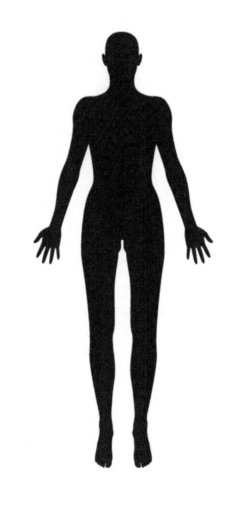

WATER   CAFFEINE   ALCOHOL

HOW I SLEPT LAST NIGHT

MOOD TRACKER

REMEMBER

My Daily Tracker

DAY

DATE

| FOOD DIARY | PHYSICAL SYMPTOMS | MEDICATIONS |

FOOD DIARY

Breakfast

Lunch

Dinner

Snacks

PHYSICAL SYMPTOMS

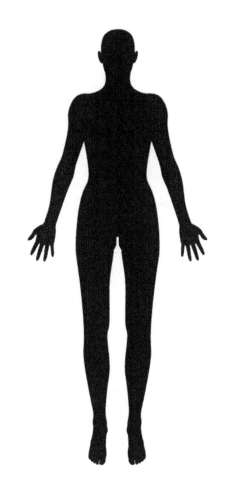

MEDICATIONS

WATER

CAFFEINE

ALCOHOL

HOW I SLEPT LAST NIGHT

MOOD TRACKER

REMEMBER

My Daily Tracker

DAY

DATE

FOOD DIARY

PHYSICAL SYMPTOMS

MEDICATIONS

Breakfast

Lunch

Dinner

Snacks

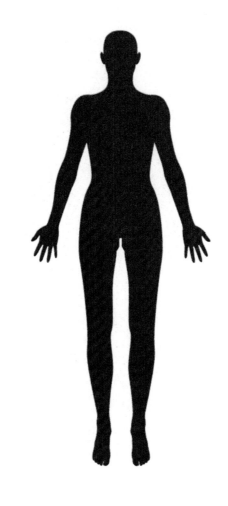

WATER
CAFFEINE
ALCOHOL

HOW I SLEPT LAST NIGHT

MOOD TRACKER

REMEMBER

My Daily Tracker

DAY

DATE

FOOD DIARY

Breakfast

Lunch

Dinner

Snacks

PHYSICAL SYMPTOMS

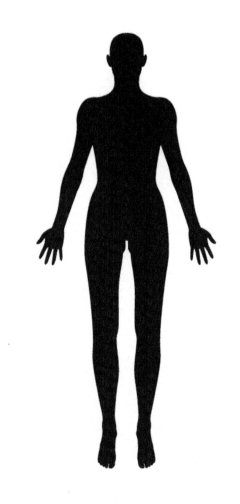

MEDICATIONS

WATER

CAFFEINE

ALCOHOL

HOW I SLEPT LAST NIGHT

MOOD TRACKER

REMEMBER

My Daily Tracker

FOOD DIARY	PHYSICAL SYMPTOMS	MEDICATIONS

Breakfast

Lunch

Dinner

Snacks

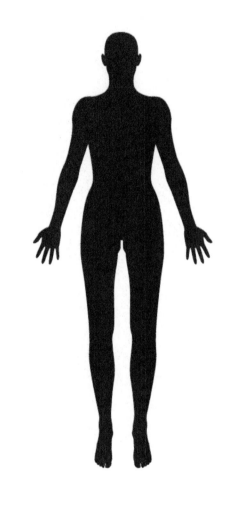

WATER   CAFFEINE   ALCOHOL   HOW I SLEPT LAST NIGHT   MOOD TRACKER

REMEMBER

My Daily Tracker

DAY

DATE

FOOD DIARY

Breakfast

Lunch

Dinner

Snacks

PHYSICAL SYMPTOMS

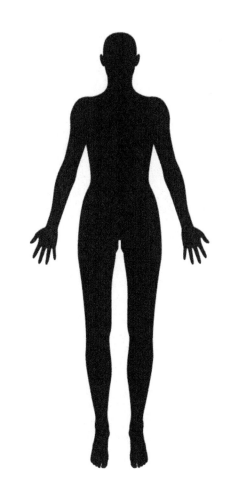

MEDICATIONS

WATER

CAFFEINE

ALCOHOL

HOW I SLEPT LAST NIGHT

MOOD TRACKER

REMEMBER

My Daily Tracker

DAY

DATE

FOOD DIARY

Breakfast

Lunch

Dinner

Snacks

PHYSICAL SYMPTOMS

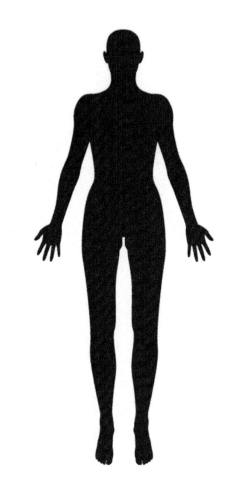

MEDICATIONS

WATER

CAFFEINE

ALCOHOL

HOW I SLEPT LAST NIGHT

MOOD TRACKER

REMEMBER

My Daily Tracker

DAY

DATE

FOOD DIARY

Breakfast

Lunch

Dinner

Snacks

PHYSICAL SYMPTOMS

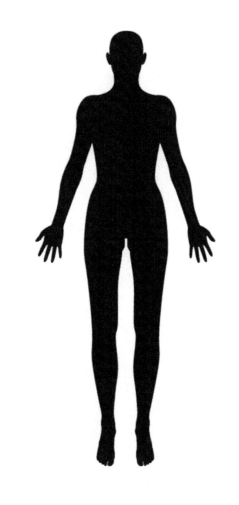

MEDICATIONS

WATER   CAFFEINE   ALCOHOL

HOW I SLEPT LAST NIGHT

MOOD TRACKER

REMEMBER

My Daily Tracker

DAY

DATE

FOOD DIARY	PHYSICAL SYMPTOMS	MEDICATIONS

Breakfast

Lunch

Dinner

Snacks

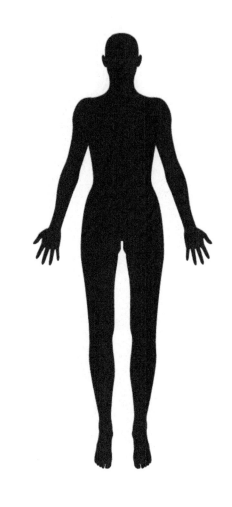

WATER   CAFFEINE   ALCOHOL

HOW I SLEPT LAST NIGHT

MOOD TRACKER

REMEMBER

My Daily Tracker

DAY

DATE

FOOD DIARY

Breakfast

Lunch

Dinner

Snacks

PHYSICAL SYMPTOMS

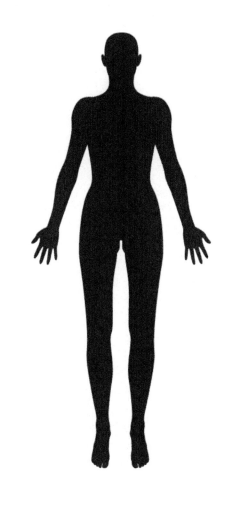

MEDICATIONS

WATER CAFFEINE ALCOHOL

HOW I SLEPT LAST NIGHT

MOOD TRACKER

REMEMBER

My Daily Tracker

FOOD DIARY	PHYSICAL SYMPTOMS	MEDICATIONS

Breakfast

Lunch

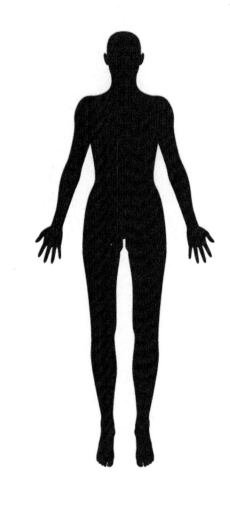

Dinner

Snacks

WATER   CAFFEINE   ALCOHOL

HOW I SLEPT LAST NIGHT

MOOD TRACKER

REMEMBER

My Daily Tracker

DAY

DATE

FOOD DIARY

Breakfast

Lunch

Dinner

Snacks

PHYSICAL SYMPTOMS

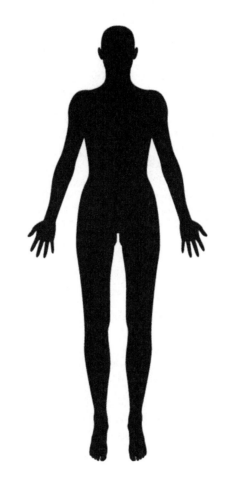

MEDICATIONS

WATER   CAFFEINE   ALCOHOL

HOW I SLEPT LAST NIGHT

MOOD TRACKER

REMEMBER

My Daily Tracker

FOOD DIARY	PHYSICAL SYMPTOMS	MEDICATIONS

Breakfast

Lunch

Dinner

Snacks

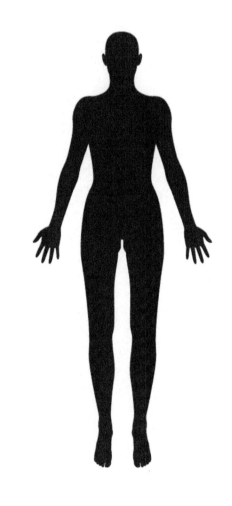

WATER	CAFFEINE	ALCOHOL	HOW I SLEPT LAST NIGHT	MOOD TRACKER

REMEMBER

My Daily Tracker

DAY

DATE

FOOD DIARY

Breakfast

Lunch

Dinner

Snacks

PHYSICAL SYMPTOMS

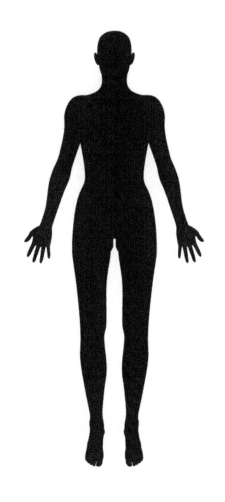

MEDICATIONS

WATER   CAFFEINE   ALCOHOL

HOW I SLEPT LAST NIGHT

MOOD TRACKER

REMEMBER

My Daily Tracker

DAY

DATE

FOOD DIARY

PHYSICAL SYMPTOMS

MEDICATIONS

Breakfast

Lunch

Dinner

Snacks

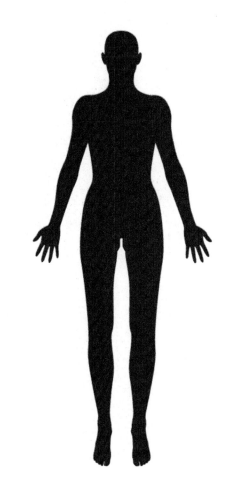

WATER

CAFFEINE

ALCOHOL

HOW I SLEPT LAST NIGHT

MOOD TRACKER

REMEMBER

My Daily Tracker

DAY

DATE

FOOD DIARY

Breakfast

Lunch

Dinner

Snacks

PHYSICAL SYMPTOMS

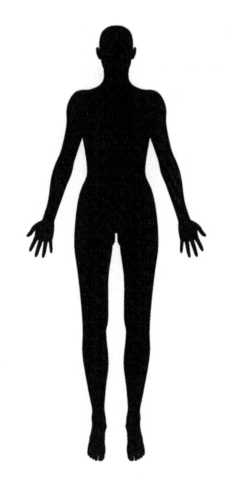

MEDICATIONS

WATER   CAFFEINE   ALCOHOL

HOW I SLEPT LAST NIGHT

MOOD TRACKER

REMEMBER

My Daily Tracker

DAY

DATE

FOOD DIARY	PHYSICAL SYMPTOMS	MEDICATIONS

Breakfast

Lunch

Dinner

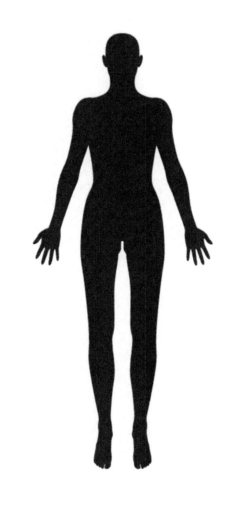

Snacks

WATER   CAFFEINE   ALCOHOL

HOW I SLEPT LAST NIGHT

MOOD TRACKER

REMEMBER

My Daily Tracker

DAY   DATE

FOOD DIARY   ## PHYSICAL SYMPTOMS   ## MEDICATIONS

Breakfast

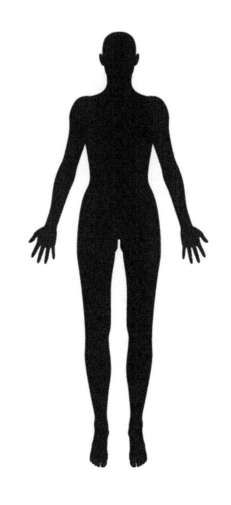

Lunch

Dinner

Snacks

WATER   CAFFEINE   ALCOHOL   HOW I SLEPT LAST NIGHT   MOOD TRACKER

REMEMBER

My Daily Tracker

DAY

DATE

FOOD DIARY

PHYSICAL SYMPTOMS

MEDICATIONS

Breakfast

Lunch

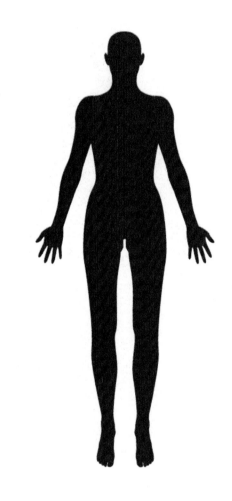

Dinner

Snacks

WATER
CAFFEINE
ALCOHOL

HOW I SLEPT LAST NIGHT

MOOD TRACKER

REMEMBER

My Daily Tracker

DAY

DATE

FOOD DIARY

Breakfast

Lunch

Dinner

Snacks

PHYSICAL SYMPTOMS

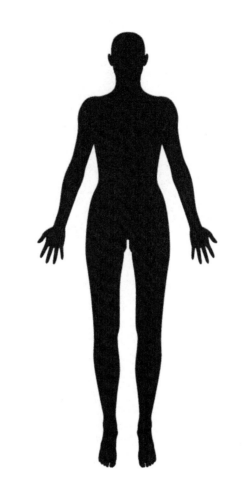

MEDICATIONS

WATER   CAFFEINE   ALCOHOL

HOW I SLEPT LAST NIGHT

MOOD TRACKER

REMEMBER

My Daily Tracker

DAY   DATE

FOOD DIARY   PHYSICAL SYMPTOMS   MEDICATIONS

Breakfast

Lunch

Dinner

Snacks

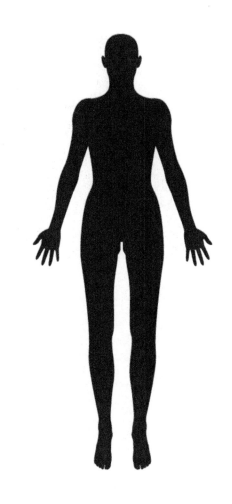

WATER   CAFFEINE   ALCOHOL   HOW I SLEPT LAST NIGHT   MOOD TRACKER

REMEMBER

My Daily Tracker

DAY

DATE

FOOD DIARY

Breakfast

Lunch

Dinner

Snacks

PHYSICAL SYMPTOMS

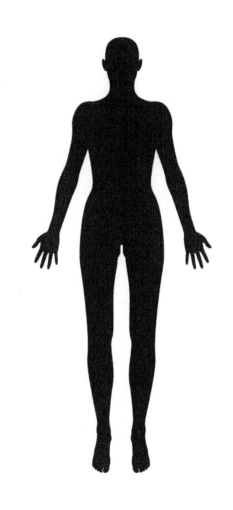

MEDICATIONS

WATER   CAFFEINE   ALCOHOL

HOW I SLEPT LAST NIGHT

MOOD TRACKER

REMEMBER

My Daily Tracker

FOOD DIARY	PHYSICAL SYMPTOMS	MEDICATIONS

Breakfast

Lunch

Dinner

Snacks

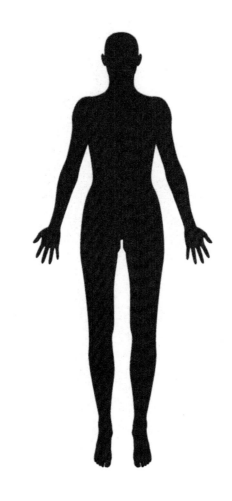

WATER	CAFFEINE	ALCOHOL

HOW I SLEPT LAST NIGHT

MOOD TRACKER

REMEMBER

My Daily Tracker

FOOD DIARY   PHYSICAL SYMPTOMS   MEDICATIONS

Breakfast

Lunch

Dinner

Snacks

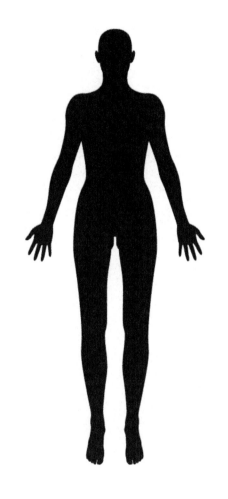

WATER   CAFFEINE   ALCOHOL

HOW I SLEPT LAST NIGHT   MOOD TRACKER

REMEMBER

My Daily Tracker

DAY

DATE

FOOD DIARY

PHYSICAL SYMPTOMS

MEDICATIONS

Breakfast

Lunch

Dinner

Snacks

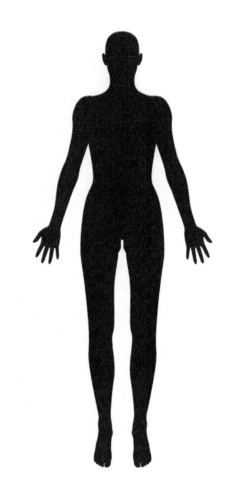

WATER   CAFFEINE   ALCOHOL

HOW I SLEPT LAST NIGHT

MOOD TRACKER

REMEMBER

My Daily Tracker

DAY

DATE

FOOD DIARY

Breakfast

Lunch

Dinner

Snacks

PHYSICAL SYMPTOMS

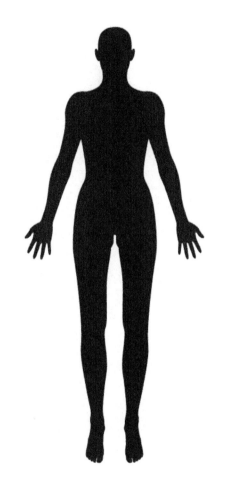

MEDICATIONS

WATER   CAFFEINE   ALCOHOL

HOW I SLEPT LAST NIGHT

MOOD TRACKER

REMEMBER

My Daily Tracker

DAY   DATE

FOOD DIARY	PHYSICAL SYMPTOMS	MEDICATIONS

Breakfast

Lunch

Dinner

Snacks

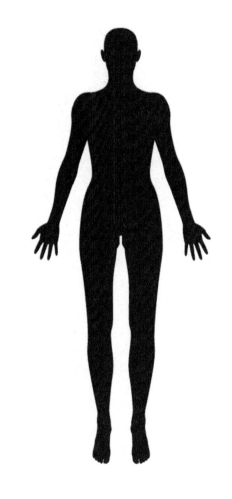

WATER   CAFFEINE   ALCOHOL

HOW I SLEPT LAST NIGHT

MOOD TRACKER

REMEMBER

My Daily Tracker

DAY

DATE

FOOD DIARY

Breakfast

Lunch

Dinner

Snacks

PHYSICAL SYMPTOMS

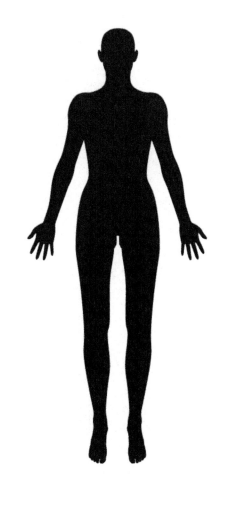

MEDICATIONS

WATER   CAFFEINE   ALCOHOL

HOW I SLEPT LAST NIGHT

MOOD TRACKER

REMEMBER

My Daily Tracker

DAY

DATE

FOOD DIARY

PHYSICAL SYMPTOMS

MEDICATIONS

Breakfast

Lunch

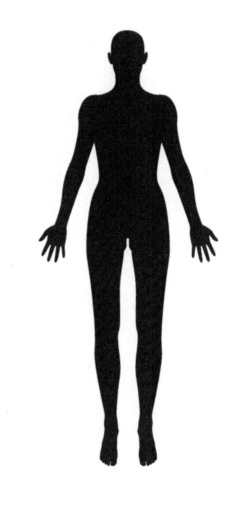

Dinner

Snacks

WATER

CAFFEINE

ALCOHOL

HOW I SLEPT LAST NIGHT

MOOD TRACKER

REMEMBER

My Daily Tracker

FOOD DIARY

Breakfast

Lunch

Dinner

Snacks

PHYSICAL SYMPTOMS

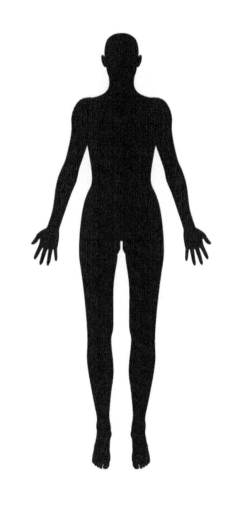

MEDICATIONS

WATER   CAFFEINE   ALCOHOL

HOW I SLEPT LAST NIGHT

MOOD TRACKER

REMEMBER

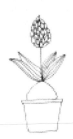
Appointment Notes
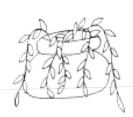

Date:

Location:

Specialist:

Contact:

Notes:

Date:

Location:

Specialist:

Contact:

Notes:

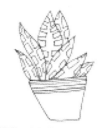

Appointment Notes

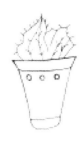

Date:

Location:

Specialist:

Contact:

Notes:

Date:

Location:

Specialist:

Contact:

Notes:

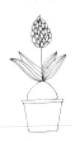

Appointment Notes

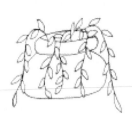

Date:

Location:

Specialist:

Contact:

Notes:

Date:

Location:

Specialist:

Contact:

Notes:

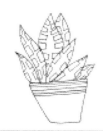

Appointment Notes

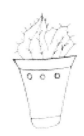

Date:

Location:

Specialist:

Contact:

Notes:

Date:

Location:

Specialist:

Contact:

Notes:

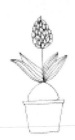

Appointment Notes

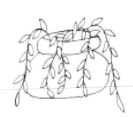

Date:

Location:

Specialist:

Contact:

Notes:

Date:

Location:

Specialist:

Contact:

Notes:

Printed in Great Britain
by Amazon